CW00481835

Yoga and Meditation

For Your Health

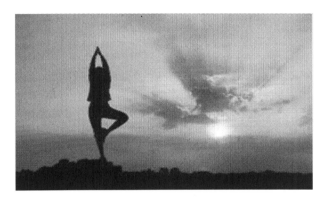

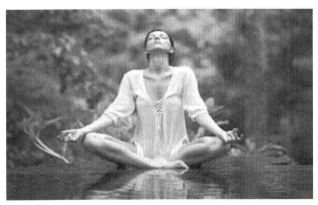

Author

Patricia Griecci

Contents

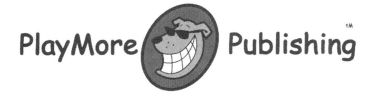

INTRODUCTION

When one mentions "yoga", many images may be conjured up. Perhaps you get an image of flower children from the 60's sitting in a circle with their legs in impossible positions chanting "Ohm" around a huge candle in a poorly lit room. Yoga is an ancient art that has been practiced for centuries. Over the years, it has risen in popularity as a way to stay fit, get in touch with one's inner self, and keep a balance of sanity in a sometimes insane world.

While yoga did come to popularity in the 60's with Maharishi Mahesh Yogi who popularized Transcendental Meditation (TM) in the 60's, because he was associated with the Beatles, yoga practitioners have brought the ancient practice to the forefront of wellness in recent years.

Many scholars believe that yoga dates back over 5,000 years to the beginning of human civilization. Scholars believe that yoga grew out of Stone Age Shamanism, because of the cultural similarities between Modern Hinduism and Mehrgarh, a neolithic settlement (in what is now Afghanistan). In fact, much of Hindu ideas, rituals and symbols of today appear to have their roots in this shamanistic culture of Mehrgahr.

Early Yoga and archaic shamanism had much in common as both sought to transcend the human condition. The primary goal of shamanism was to heal members of the community and act as religious mediators. Archaic Yoga was also community oriented, as it attempted to discern the cosmic order through inner vision, then to apply that order to daily living. Later, Yoga evolved into a more inward experience, and Yogis focused on their individual enlightenment and salvation.

Yoga is the most diversified spiritual practice in the world. Crossing over many cultures (including Hinduism, Buddhism, Jainism and the West), Yoga also extends over multiple languages such as Hindi, Tibetan, Bengali, Sanskrit, Tamil, Prakit, Marathi and Pali. The Yogic tradition continues to proliferate and spread its message of peace to this very day.

There are many different places that offer yoga classes – gyms, wellness centers, even the local YMCA. But you don't have to join a class to practice yoga. It is just as easily done in your home or even at your desk while at work. Yoga can help bring you inner peace when you are stressed out. It can even help relieve the pain of headaches, backaches, and menstrual cramps.

As studies continue to reveal yoga's many health benefits, this centuries- old Eastern philosophy is fast becoming the new fitness soul mate for workout enthusiasts.

Contemporary devotees range from high-powered execs trying to keep hearts beating on a healthy note to image-conscious Hollywood stars striving for sleek physiques. Even prominent athletes are adding yoga to their training regime to develop balanced, injury-free muscles and spines.

Yet to applaud yoga for its physical benefits alone would only diminish what this entire system has to offer as a whole. By practicing yoga on a regular basis, you may be surprised to find that you're building much more than a strong, flexible body.

Initially, the sole purpose of practicing yoga was to experience spiritual enlightenment. In Sanskrit (the ancient language of India), yoga translates as "yoke" or "union," describing the integration of mind and body to create a greater connection with one's own pure, essential nature.

Classes that have gained popularity in the United States usually teach one of the many types of hatha yoga, a physical discipline which focuses mainly on asanas (postures) and breath work in order to prepare the body for spiritual pursuits.

We will attempt to simplify the ancient practice of yoga by showing you some basic yoga positions, giving you tips on performing yoga exercises, and inducting meditation practices into your everyday life. Through yoga and meditation, you could come to a new level of enlightenment with your personal life and enhance the quality of your existence.

No longer is yoga a mysterious phenomenon. It is now simply a way to keep you healthy and aligned. Now relax and read on as we explore yoga and meditation.

WHAT IS YOGA?

As we have said, yoga is an ancient Indian philosophy that enhances personal growth and well-being. Although it is a systemic philosophical approach, yoga is not a religion, but complementary with most spiritual paths.

The physical aspect of Yoga (Hatha Yoga) use poses and focused breathing, requiring concentration and discipline. The result is a greater union of mind, body and spirit. Anyone, regardless or body type, age, experience, or physical abilities, can practice yoga.

Pop culture would have us believe that yoga involves contorting your body into uncomfortable positions while staring at a candle and breathing incense. You will see that yoga is much more than that. It is a series of exercises that can be done by almost all people – not just the young who are in shape and healthy. Yoga can be performed by senior citizens, disabled people, and even children.

Yoga is a tool for gaining body-mind awareness to enhance whatever spiritual/religious beliefs you have.

A yoga session will leave you feeling energized and relaxed. You will work your muscles and will properly align your bones; you will breathe deeply, oxygenating the lungs and blood; you will experience true deep relaxation.

By bringing awareness to the body, and working the muscles, you are able to more deeply relax them than from any other form of exercise. You will gain a deeper appreciation of your body and mind through yoga in a way that no other exercise program will.

People who have done no physical exercise at all, as well as Olympic athletes, find enormous benefits from Yoga. The foundation of traditional yoga is careful alignment of your body as you hold the poses. This precision and the awareness that comes with it, leads to tremendous growth, physically, mentally, and emotionally.

As in all great arts and sciences, to become proficient in yoga requires effort, determination, and practice. But then, the fruit we reap is always in proportion to the seeds we sow and nurture. Thus, if you are looking for a quick fix, an instant cure, a quelling of surface symptoms while the true ailment remains unhealed, you will not find satisfaction in yoga.

On the other hand, if you want to keep or regain your health, vitality and vigor; if you want to feel younger and stronger; and if you are looking for a perfectly balanced and complete form of exercise that can be started by anyone over seven years of age, in any condition, and which becomes more challenging as you get more advanced, yoga is for you!

There are many benefits of a regular yoga practice. Not only does yoga help maintain a healthy lifestyle, it clears your mind and provide clarity of focus – something we all could use from time to time! Let's look at the benefits of yoga.

WHY DO YOGA?

Yoga Creates both flexibility and strength along with cardiovascular health. It creates mental clarity and focus and emotional balance. Yoga is safe for all ages and body types. It facilitates healing from injuries and is a wonderful way to create wellness.

You weight train to gain strength, jog or do aerobics for a cardiovascular workout, practice tai-chi to develop a sense of balance and harmony, stretch to gain flexibility, and meditate to develop peace of mind and relaxation. Yoga is a form of exercise that gives you everything: strength, endurance, balance, flexibility, and relaxation.

It is the only complete form of bodywork that does it all. Indeed, yoga is more than stretching and relaxation: it is the ultimate mind- body challenge.

Yoga increases flexibility as it offers positions that act upon the various joints of the body including those joints that aren't always in the forefront of notice ability. These joints are rarely exercised, however, with yoga, they are!

Various yoga positions exercise the different tendons and ligaments of the body. The body that may have been quite rigid begins experiencing a remarkable flexibility in even those parts which have not been consciously worked upon. Seemingly unrelated non-strenuous yoga positions act upon certain parts of the body in an interrelated manner. When done together, they work in harmony to create a situation where flexibility is attained relatively easily.

Yoga is perhaps the only form of activity which massages all the internal glands and organs of the body in a thorough manner, including those – such as the prostate - that hardly get externally stimulated during our entire lifetime. Yoga acts in a wholesome manner on the various body parts. This stimulation and massage of the organs in turn benefits us by keeping away disease and providing a forewarning at the first possible instance of a likely onset of disease or disorder.

By gently stretching muscles and joints as well as massaging the various organs, yoga ensures the optimum blood supply to various parts of the body. This helps in the flushing out of toxins from every nook and cranny as well as providing nourishment up to the last point. This leads to benefits such as delayed ageing, energy and a remarkable zest for life.

But these enormous physical benefits are just a "side effect" of this powerful practice. What yoga does is harmonize the mind with the body. This results in real quantum benefits. It is now an open secret that the will of the mind has enabled people to achieve extraordinary physical feats, which proves beyond doubt the mind and body connection.

Yoga through meditation works remarkably to achieve this harmony and helps the mind work in sync with the body. How often do we find that we are unable to perform our activities properly and in a satisfying manner because of the confusions and conflicts in our mind weigh down heavily upon us? Moreover, stress which in reality is the #1 killer affecting all parts of our physical, endocrinal and emotional systems can be corrected through the wonderful yoga practice of meditation.

In fact yoga = meditation, because both work together in achieving the common goal of unity of mind, body and spirit – a state of eternal bliss.

The meditative practices through yoga help in achieving an emotional balance through detachment. What it means is that meditation creates conditions, where you are not affected by the happenings around you. This in turn creates a remarkable calmness and a positive outlook, which also has tremendous benefits on the physical health of the body.

There's no doubt that yoga has tremendous benefits to your health and well-being. So how do you get started with your own yoga program? Let's look at the basic styles of yoga and what they mean.

WHICH IS RIGHT FOR YOU?

In ancient times yoga was often referred to as a tree, a living entity with roots, a trunk, branches, blossoms, and fruit. Hatha yoga is one of six branches; the others include raja, karma, bhakti, jnana, and tantra yoga. Each branch with its unique characteristics and function represents a particular approach to life. Some people may find one particular branch more inviting than another. However, it is important to note that involvement in one of these paths does not preclude activity in any of the others, and in fact you'll find many paths naturally overlapping.

Raja Yoga

Raja means "royal," and meditation is the focal point of this branch of yoga. This approach involves strict adherence to the eight "limbs" of yoga as outlined by Patanajli in the Yoga Sutras. Also found in many other branches of yoga, these limbs, or stages, follow this order: ethical standards, yama; self-discipline, niyama; posture, asana; breath extension or control, pranayama; sensory withdrawl, pratyahara; concentration, dharana; meditation, dhyana; and ecstasy or final liberation, samadhi.

Raja yoga attracts individuals who are introspective and drawn to meditation. Members of religious orders and spiritual communities devote themselves to this branch of yoga. However, even though this path suggests a monastic or contemplative lifestyle, entering an ashram or monastery is not a prerequisite to practicing raja yoga.

Karma Yoga

The next branch is that of karma yoga or the path of service, and none of us can escape this pathway. The principle of karma yoga is that what we experience today is created by our actions in the past. Being aware of this, all of our present efforts become a way to consciously create a future that frees us from being bound by negativity and selfishness.

Karma is the path of self-transcending action.

We practice karma yoga whenever we perform our work and live our lives in a selfless fashion and as a way to serve others. Volunteering to serve meals in a soup kitchen or signing up for a stint with the Peace Corps or Habitat for Humanity are prime examples of selfless service associated with the karma yoga path.

Bhakti Yoga

Bhakti yoga describes the path of devotion. Seeing the divine in all of creation, bhakti yoga is a positive way to channel the emotions. The path of bhakti provides us with an opportunity to cultivate acceptance and tolerance for everyone we come into contact with.

Bhakti yogis express the devotional nature of their path in their every thought, word, and deed—whether they are taking out the trash or calming the anger of a loved one. Mahatma Gandhi and Martin Luther King, Jr., are prime examples of bhakti yogis. The life and work of Mother Teresa epitomize the combination of the karma and bhakti yoga paths with devotional aspects of bhakti and the selfless service of karma yoga.

Jnana Yoga

If we consider bhakti to be the yoga of the heart, then jnana yoga is the yoga of the mind, of wisdom, the path of the sage or scholar. This path requires development of the intellect through the study of the scriptures and texts of the yogic tradition.

The jnana yoga approach is considered the most difficult and at the same time the most direct. It involves serious study and will appeal to those who are more intellectually inclined. Within the context of our Western religious traditions, Kabalistic scholars, Jesuit priests, and Benedictine monks epitomize jnana yogis.

Tantra Yoga

Probably the most misunderstood or misinterpreted of all the yogas, tantra, the sixth branch, is the pathway of ritual, which includes consecrated sexuality. The key word here is "consecrated," which means to make sacred, to set apart as something holy or hallowed.

In tantric practice we experience the Divine in everything we do. A reverential attitude is therefore cultivated, encouraging a ritualistic approach to life. It is amusing to note that, although tantra has become associated exclusively with sexual ritual, most tantric schools actually recommend a celibate lifestyle.

In essence, tantra is the most esoteric of the six major branches. It will appeal to those yogis who enjoy ceremony and relate to the feminine principle of the cosmos, which yogis call shakti.

If you see—and are deeply moved by—the significance behind celebration and ritual (holidays, birthdays, anniversaries, and other rites of passage), tantra yoga may be for you.

Many tantric yogis find magic in all types of ceremony, whether it be a Japanese tea ceremony, the consecration of the Eucharist in a Catholic mass, or the consummation of a relationship.

ASHTANGA YOGA

One of the most popular schools of yoga practice today is that of Ashtanga Yoga. Ashtanga literally means "eight limbs". These eight steps (limbs) basically act as guidelines on how to live a meaningful and purposeful life. They serve as a prescription for moral and ethical conduct and self-discipline; they direct attention toward one's health; and they help us to acknowledge the spiritual aspects of our nature.

The first limb, yama, deals with one's ethical standards and sense of integrity, focusing on our behavior and how we conduct ourselves in life. Yamas are universal practices that relate best to what we know as the Golden Rule, "Do unto others as you would have them do unto you."

Niyama, the second limb, has to do with self-discipline and spiritual observances. Regularly attending temple or church services, saying grace before meals, developing your own personal meditation practices, or making a habit of taking contemplative walks alone are all examples of niyamas in practice.

Asanas, the postures practiced in yoga, comprise the third limb. In the yogic view, the body is a temple of spirit, the care of which is an important stage of our spiritual growth.

Through the practice of asanas, we develop the habit of discipline and the ability to concentrate, both of which are necessary for meditation.

Generally translated as breath control, this fourth stage consists of techniques designed to gain mastery over the respiratory process while recognizing the connection between the breath, the mind, and the emotions.

As implied by the literal translation of pranayama, "life force extension," yogis believe that it not only rejuvenates the body but actually extends life itself. You can practice pranayama as an isolated technique (i.e., simply sitting and performing a number of breathing exercises), or integrate it into your daily hatha yoga routine.

These first four stages of Patanjali's ashtanga yoga concentrate on refining our personalities, gaining mastery over the body, and developing an energetic awareness of ourselves, all of which prepares us for the second half of this journey, which deals with the senses, the mind, and attaining a higher state of consciousness.

Pratyahara, the fifth limb, means withdrawal or sensory transcendence.
It is during this stage that we make the conscious effort to draw our awareness away from the external world and outside stimuli.

Keenly aware of, yet cultivating a detachment from, our senses, we direct our attention internally.

The practice of pratyahara provides us with an opportunity to step back and take a look at ourselves. This withdrawal allows us to objectively observe our cravings: habits that are perhaps detrimental to our health and which likely interfere with our inner growth.

As each stage prepares us for the next, the practice of pratyahara creates the setting for dharana, or concentration. Having relieved ourselves of outside distractions, we can now deal with the distractions of the mind itself. No easy task!

In the practice of concentration, which precedes meditation, we learn how to slow down the thinking process by concentrating on a single mental object: a specific energetic center in the body, an image of a deity, or the silent repetition of a sound. We, of course, have already begun to develop our powers of concentration in the previous three stages of posture, breath control, and withdrawal of the senses.

In asana and pranayama, although we pay attention to our actions, our attention travels. Our focus constantly shifts as we fine-tune the many nuances of any particular posture or breathing technique.

In pratyahara we become self- observant; now, in dharana, we focus our attention on a single point. Extended periods of concentration naturally lead to meditation.

Meditation or contemplation, the seventh stage of ashtanga, is the uninterrupted flow of concentration. Although concentration (dharana) and meditation (dhyana) may appear to be one and the same, a fine line of distinction exists between these two stages. Where dharana practices one-pointed attention, dhyana is ultimately a state of being keenly aware without focus.

At this stage, the mind has been quieted, and in the stillness it produces few or no thoughts at all. The strength and stamina it takes to reach this state of stillness is quite impressive. But don't give up. While this may seem a difficult if not impossible task, remember that yoga is a process. Even though we may not attain the "picture perfect" pose, or the ideal state of consciousness, we benefit at every stage of our progress.

Patanjali describes this eighth and final stage of ashtanga as a state of ecstasy. At this stage, the meditator merges with his or her point of focus and transcends the Self altogether. The meditator comes to realize a profound connection to the Divine, interconnectedness with all living things. With this realization comes the "peace that passeth all understanding"; the experience of bliss and being at one with the Universe.

On the surface, this may seem to be a rather lofty, "holier than thou" kind of goal. However, if we pause to examine what we really want to get out of life, would not joy, fulfillment, and freedom somehow find their way onto our list of hopes, wishes, and desires?

What Patanjali has described as the completion of the yogic path is what, deep down, all human beings aspire to: peace. We also might give some thought to the fact that this ultimate stage of yoga—enlightenment—can neither be bought nor possessed. It can only be experienced, the price of which is the continual devotion of the aspirant

OK, now that we've got that out of the way, let's prep the environment and get you ready for your yoga workout!

GETTING READY

Now that you've decided to take up yoga for your health, you must consider the best environment and preparation to do so.

The very best time to practice yoga is first thing in the morning before breakfast. Upon waking, empty the bowels, shower if you wish, then commence the day with your regime of yoga practices. The second most conducive time is early evening, around sunset.

It is, of course, far better to do something at a time of the day which suits one, rather than to miss out by being too rigid or idealistic. Always remember integral yoga is a balanced recipe which maintains that to get the best from your yoga practice, you should whenever possible, mix and match the necessary elements of practice which will improve and enhance your spiritual growth and awareness.

Asanas – yoga postures - may be practiced at any time of day except within 2-3 hours of having eaten. You can do postures when the body feels stiff, tense, tired or hyped-up. Be aware not to do too many over-stimulating postures just before bedtime. Asanas are best practiced first in your yoga routine, followed by breathing (Pranayama) and then meditation.

Pranayama may be practiced at any time of day except within 2-3 hours after meals. It may be done when tense or tired or when space does not allow room for postures. Pranayama is best practiced straight after asanas without breaking the flow of awareness. Pranayama is a necessary pre-requisite for successful meditation.

Meditation may be done at any time of day when you feel both awake and relaxed. For best results, you should not do meditation within 2-3 hours of eating, when sleepy, or when mentally "hyped-up".

It is best is to have fresh air in a quiet and clean place that suits the concentration and awareness yoga will create. Do not practice yoga in direct sunlight or after sun-bathing. Outdoors is OK but you should avoid cold wind and insects. Wear loose comfortable yoga clothing so there is no restriction around the limbs.

Exercise on an empty stomach at least three hours after eating.

Do not force your body under any circumstances. Many people don't take heed of this advice. They try to push their bodies into the exercises, whether the body is ready or not. This is a great mistake which does more harm than you can imagine.

Work slowly with your body. Respect its limits. These limits will gradually extend and you will gain flexibility if you work regularly and sensitively at stretching your limits. The body will get the message and the tension which is preventing   you from   proceeding   will   gradually   be   released. Relax briefly between each practice. Remember the golden rule: "If it's uncomfortable – DON'T"

Do not continue any exercise which causes pain. Pain is a message from the body which must be listened to. In some cases it may simply be the body's process of changing. In such cases, you simply need to bear with it and continue (without forcing) and it will gradually pass.

In other cases you may be doing harm to some part of your body and may have to stop and do some other preparatory exercises before returning to that one. Check with your doctor or other professional if you have concerns.

Be conscientious and concentrate on what you are doing. Keep your mind on feeling what is happening in the body and concentrate on your breath and position. Do not think about other things or talk to anyone while exercising. If possible, it would be best if you were alone in the room, without distractions such as radio or TV, so that you can concentrate. If this is not possible, just try to concentrate on yourself and ignore what is going on around you.

Give importance to your breathing. Each exercise has a specific way of breathing. This is an extremely important aspect of the exercise. In many cases, it is even more important than the physical movements themselves. Be conscious of your breathing and breathe slowly and deeply, according to the instructions for each exercise. In general (with some exceptions) we inhale when we stretch upward or backward and exhale when we bend downward or forward. Always breathe through the nose both in and out, unless specified otherwise. Remember "Nose for breathing-mouth for eating".

Allow your attention to flow through the body as you become aware of each muscle and the tension and energy stored there and allow that energy to flow and the muscle relax.   Complete your exercise series with deep breathing and, if possible, with deep relaxation.

There are no age limits either young or old for the practice of yoga. However the application of the techniques will vary according to the abilities of the practitioner.   Those with disabilities, severe, acute or chronic medical conditions should consult both with their medical practitioner and their yoga teacher to assess any dangers or difficulties which may arise.

Avoid exercising at least three months after surgery, unless you have specific permission from your doctor. Some exercises should be resumed only 6 months after surgery, unless you have your doctor's permission to start earlier.

Also, avoid all exercises at any time when you suspect internal bleeding or an inflamed appendix.

Never practice any yoga techniques under the influence of alcohol or mind altering drugs.   There are no hard and fast dietary rules necessary to begin the practice of yoga. One does not have to give up smoking, become vegetarian, or be a purist to learn yoga.

What you might find, however, is that yoga can help you overcome those bad habits you've been wanting to shed for years and bring you into alignment with your spiritual side which can be key to overcoming vices.

Now let's look at some of the asanas, or positions, that are central to a yoga regime. We'll give you a good basic beginning yoga workout to begin your journey!

BEGINNING YOUR WORKOUT

We use the word "workout" loosely here because, as we've pointed out, yoga is less workout and more mind-body exploration. Workout implies sweating as you push your body into exercise mode. That isn't what yoga is about.

So, here's a good way to start your yoga plan. Do these exercises in the order given for a good beginning workout.

EasyPose

Begin with the easy pose. Easy pose is a comfortable seated position for meditation. This pose opens the hips, lengthens the spine and promotes grounding and inner calm. Basically, you're sitting cross legged like you did in school as a young child. "Criss cross apple sauce", as my teacher used to say!

With the buttocks on the floor, cross your legs and place your feet directly below your knees. Rest your hands on your knees with the palms facing up.

Press your hip bones down into the floor and reach the crown of the head up to lengthen the spine. Drop your shoulders down and back and press your chest towards the front of the room.

Relax your face, jaw, and belly. Let your tongue rest on the roof of your mouth just behind your front teeth. Breathe deeply through the nose down into the belly and hold as long as is comfortable.

Downward-FacingDog

After the easy pose, move into downward-facing dog. This is one of the most widely recognized yoga poses. Downward-Facing Dog is an all-over, rejuvenating stretch.

Benefits include:

Calms the brain and helps relieve stress and mild depression

Energizes the body

Stretches the shoulders, hamstrings, calves, arches, and hands

Strengthens the arms and legs

Helps relieve the symptoms of menopause

Relieves menstrual discomfort when done with head supported

Helps prevent osteoporosis

Improves digestion

Relieves headache, insomnia, back pain, and fatigue

Therapeutic for high blood pressure, asthma, flat feet, sciatica, sinusitis

Use caution doing this pose if you have carpal tunnel syndrome, are in the late stages of pregnancy, or suffer from high blood pressure.

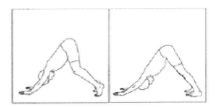

Come onto the floor on your hands and knees. Set your knees directly below your hips and your hands slightly forward of your shoulders. Spread your palms, index fingers parallel or slightly turned out, and turn your toes under.

Exhale and lift your knees away from the floor. At first keep the knees slightly bent and the heels lifted away from the floor. Lengthen your tailbone away from the back of your pelvis and press it lightly toward the pubis. Against this resistance, lift the sitting bones toward the ceiling, and from your inner ankles draw the inner legs up into the groins.

Then with an exhalation, push your top thighs back and stretch your heels onto or down toward the floor. Straighten your knees but be sure not to lock them. Firm the outer thighs and roll the upper thighs inward slightly. Narrow the front of the pelvis.

Firm the outer arms and press the bases of the index fingers actively into the floor. From these two points, lift along your inner arms from the wrists to the tops of the shoulders. Firm your shoulder blades against your back then widen them and draw them toward the tailbone. Keep the head between the upper arms; don't let it hang.

Stay in this pose anywhere from 1 to 3 minutes. Then bend your knees to the floor with an exhalation and rest.

SunSalutations

On days when you think you have no time for yoga, try and do at least one or two rounds of the Sun Salutation. You'll feel the difference.

After downward-facing dog, move into 3 rounds of sun salutations.

Stand facing the direction of the sun with both feet touching. Bring the hands together, palm-to-palm, at the heart. Inhale and raise the arms upward. Slowly bend backward, stretching arms above the head. Exhale slowly bending forward, touching the earth with respect until the hands are in line with the feet, head touching knees.

Inhale and move the right leg back away from the body in a wide backward step. Keep the hands and feet firmly on the ground, with the left foot between the hands. Raise the head. While exhaling, bring the left foot together with the right.

Keep arms straight, raise the hips and align the head with the arms, forming an upward arch. Exhale and lower the body to the floor until the feet, knees, hands, chest, and forehead are touching the ground. Inhale and slowly raise the head and bend backward as much as possible, bending the spine to the maximum

While exhaling, bring the left foot together with the right. Keep arms straight, raise the hips and align the head with the arms, forming an upward arch. Inhale and move the right leg back away from the body in a wide backward step.

Keep the hands and feet firmly on the ground, with the left foot between the hands. Raise the head.   Exhale slowly bending forward, touching the earth with respect until the hands are in line with the feet, head touching knees.

Inhale and raise the arms upward. Slowly bend backward, stretching arms above the head.   Stand facing the direction of the sun with both feet touching. Bring the hands together, palm-to-palm, at the heart.

The sequence will look something like this:

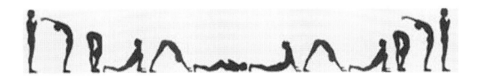

TreePose-VrikshaAsana

Benefits include:

Strengthens thighs, calves, ankles, and spine

Stretches the groins and inner thighs, chest and shoulders

Improves sense of balance

Relieves sciatica and reduces flat feet

Use caution if you suffer from insomnia or low blood pressure. If you have high blood pressure, do not raise your arms above your head.

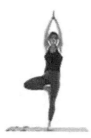

Stand with the feet together and the arms by your sides. Bend the right leg at the knee, raise the right thigh and bring the sole of the right foot as high up the inside of the left thigh as possible.

Balancing on the left foot, raise both arms over the head, keep the elbows unbent and join the palms together.

Hold the posture while breathing gently through the nostrils for about 10 complete breaths.

Lower the arms and right leg and return to the tad-asana, standing position with feet together and arms at the sides. Pause for a few moments and repeat on the opposite leg. Do this two or three times per leg or as long as is comfortable.

The challenge of the vriksha-asana is maintaining balance on one leg. Poor balance is often the result of a restless mind or distracted attention. Regular practice of this posture will help focus the mind and cultivate concentration (dharana).

When practicing vriksha-asana it may help to imagine or picture a tree in the mind and apply the following technique: Imagine that the foot you are balanced on is the root of the tree and the leg is the trunk.

Continue by imagining the head and outstretched arms as the branches and leaves of the tree. You may be unsteady for a while and find the body swaying back and forth, but don't break the concentration. Like a tree bending in the wind and yet remaining upright, the body can maintain balance.

Aim to achieve the "rootedness" and firmness of a tree. Regular practice of the vriksha-asana improves concentration, balance and coordination.

Because the weight of the entire body is balanced on one foot, the muscles of that leg are strengthened and toned as well.

As you advance in this posture and are able to remain standing for more than a few moments, try closing the eyes and maintaining your balance.

ExtendedTrianglePose

Benefits include:
Stretches and strengthens the thighs, knees, and ankles

Stretches the hips, groins, hamstrings, and calves; shoulders, chest, and spine

Stimulates the abdominal organs

Helps relieve stress

Improves digestion

Helps relieve the symptoms of menopause

Relieves backache, especially through second trimester of pregnancy

Therapeutic for anxiety, flat feet, infertility, neck pain, osteoporosis, and sciatica.

Use caution if you suffer from low blood pressure, have a heart condition, or have neck problems.

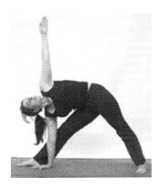

Stand with the feet together and the arms by your sides. Separate the feet slightly further than shoulder distance apart. Inhale and raise both arms straight out from the shoulders parallel to the floor with the palms facing down.

Exhale slowly while turning the torso to the left, bend at the waist and bring the right hand down to the left ankle. The palm of the right hand is placed along the outside of the left ankle. The left arm should be extended upward. Both legs and arms are kept straight without bending the knees and elbows.

Turn the head upward to the left and gaze up at the fingertips of the left hand. Inhale and return to a standing position with the arms outstretched.

Hold this position for the duration of the exhaled breath. Exhale and repeat on the opposite side.

The triangle pose is basically doing slow toe touches while concentrating on your breathing and stretching your body.

SeatedForwardBend–Paschimottanasana

Literally translated as "intense stretch of the west," Paschimottanasana can help a distracted mind unwind.

Benefits include:

Calms the brain and helps relieve stress and mild depression

Stretches the spine, shoulders, hamstrings Stimulates the liver, kidneys, ovaries, and uterus Improves digestion
Helps relieve the symptoms of menopause and menstrual discomfort

Soothes headache and anxiety and reduces fatigue

Therapeutic for high blood pressure, infertility, insomnia, and sinusitis

Traditional texts say that Paschimottanasana increases appetite, reduces obesity, and cures diseases.

Use caution if you suffer from asthma or have a back injury.

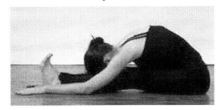

Sit on the floor with your buttocks supported on a folded blanket and your legs straight in front of you. Press actively through your heels. Rock slightly onto your left buttock, and pull your right sitting bone away from the heel with your right hand. Repeat on the other side.

Turn the top thighs in slightly and press them down into the floor. Press through your palms or finger tips on the floor beside your hips and lift the top of the sternum toward the ceiling as the top thighs descend.

Draw the inner groins deep into the pelvis. Inhale, and keeping the front torso long, lean forward from the hip joints, not the waist. Lengthen the tailbone away from the back of your pelvis. If possible take the sides of the feet with your hands, thumbs on the soles, elbows fully extended; if this isn't possible, loop a strap around the foot soles, and hold the strap firmly. Be sure your elbows are straight, not bent.

When you are ready to go further, don't forcefully pull yourself into the forward bend, whether your hands are on the feet or holding the strap.

Always lengthen the front torso into the pose, keeping your head raised.

If you are holding the feet, bend the elbows out to the sides and lift them away from the floor; if holding the strap, lighten your grip and walk the hands forward, keeping the arms long. The lower belly should touch the thighs first, and then the upper belly, then the ribs, and the head last.

With each inhalation, lift and lengthen the front torso just slightly; with each exhalation release a little more fully into the forward bend. In this way the torso oscillates and lengthens almost imperceptibly with the breath. Eventually you may be able to stretch the arms out beyond the feet on the floor.

Stay in the pose anywhere from 1 to 3 minutes. To come up, first lift the torso away from the thighs and straighten the elbows again if they are bent. Then inhale and lift the torso up by pulling the tailbone down and into the pelvis.

BoundAnglePose-BaddhaKonasana

Bound Angle Pose, also called Cobbler's Pose after the typical sitting position of Indian cobblers, is an excellent groin and hip-opener.

Benefits include:

Stimulates abdominal organs, ovaries and prostate gland, bladder, and kidneys

Stimulates the heart and improves general circulation

Stretches the inner thighs, groins, and knees

Helps relieve mild depression, anxiety, and fatigue

Soothes menstrual discomfort and sciatica

Helps relieve the symptoms of menopause

Therapeutic for flat feet, high blood pressure, infertility, and asthma

Consistent practice of this pose until late into pregnancy is said to help ease childbirth.

Traditional texts say that Baddha Konasana destroys disease and gets rid of fatigue.

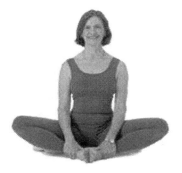

Sit with your legs straight out in front of you, raising your pelvis on a blanket if your hips or groins are tight. Exhale, bend your knees, pull your heels toward your pelvis, then drop your knees out to the sides and press the soles of your feet together.

Bring your heels as close to your pelvis as you comfortably can. With the first and second finger and thumb, grasp the big toe of each foot. Always keep the outer edges of the feet firmly on the floor. If it isn't possible to hold the toes, clasp each hand around the same-side ankle or shin.

Sit so that the pubis in front and the tailbone in back are equidistant from the floor. The perineum then will be approximately parallel to the floor and the pelvis in a neutral position. Firm the sacrum and shoulder blades against the back and lengthen the front torso through the top of the sternum.

Never force your knees down. Instead release the heads of the thigh bones toward the floor. When this action leads, the knees follow.
Stay in this pose anywhere from 1 to 5 minutes. Then inhale, lift your knees away from the floor, and extend the legs back to their original position.

Upavistha Konasana is a good preparation for most of the seated forward bends and twists, as well as the wide-leg standing poses

Benefits include:

Stretches the insides and backs of the legs Stimulates the abdominal organs Strengthens the spine
Calms the brain

Releases groins

Use caution with this exercise if you have a lower back injury.

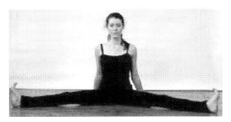

Sit with your legs extended out in front of you, then lean your torso back slightly on your hands and lift and open your legs to an angle of about 90 degrees (the legs should form an approximate right angle, with the pubis at the apex).
Press your hands against the floor and slide your buttocks forward, widening the legs another 10 to 20 degrees. If you can't sit comfortably on the floor, raise your buttocks on a folded blanket.

Rotate your thighs outwardly, pinning the outer thighs against the floor, so that the knee caps point straight up toward the ceiling. Reach out through your heels and stretch your soles, pressing though the balls of the feet.

With your thigh bones pressed heavily into the floor and your knee caps pointing up at the ceiling, walk your hands forward between your legs. Keep your arms long.

As with all forward bends, the emphasis is on moving from the hip joints and maintaining the length of the front torso. As soon as you find yourself bending from the waist, stop, re-establish the length from the pubis to the navel, and continue forward if possible.

Increase the forward bend on each exhalation until you feel a comfortable stretch in the backs of your legs. Stay in the pose 1 minute or longer. Then come up on an inhalation with a long front torso.

FullBoatPose

An abdominal and deep hip flexor strengthener,
Boat Pose requires you to balance on the tripod of your sitting bones and tailbone.

Benefits include:

Strengthens the abdomen, hip flexors, and spine

Stimulates the kidneys, thyroid and prostate glands, and intestines

Helps relieve stress

Improves digestion

Use caution if you have low blood pressure, insomnia, neck problems, are pregnant or menstruating.

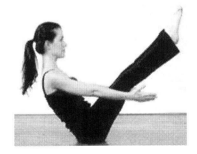

Sit on the floor with your legs straight in front of you. Press your hands on the floor a little behind your hips, fingers pointing toward the feet, and strengthen the arms. Lift through the top of the sternum and lean back slightly.

As you do this make sure your back doesn't round; continue to lengthen the front of your torso between the pubis and top sternum. Sit on the "tripod" of your two sitting bones and tailbone.

Exhale and bend your knees, then lift your feet off the floor, so that the thighs are angled about 45-50 degrees relative to the floor. Lengthen your tailbone into the floor and lift your pubis toward your navel. If possible, slowly straighten your knees, raising the tips of your toes slightly above the level of your eyes. If this isn't possible remain with your knees bent, perhaps lifting the shins parallel to the floor.

Stretch your arms alongside the legs, parallel to each other and the floor. Spread the shoulder blades across your back and reach strongly out through the fingers. If this isn't possible, keep the hands on the floor beside your hips or hold on to the backs of your thighs.

While the lower belly should be firm, it shouldn't get hard and thick. Try to keep the lower belly relatively flat. Press the heads of the thigh bones toward the floor to help anchor the pose and lift the top sternum. Breathe easily. Tip the chin slightly toward the sternum so the base of the skull lifts lightly away from the back of the neck.

At first stay in the pose for 10-20 seconds. Gradually increase the time of your stay to 1 minute.
Release the legs with an exhalation and sit upright on an inhalation.

BridgePose

This active version of Bridge Pose calms the brain and rejuvenates tired
legs.

Benefits include:

Stretches the chest, neck, and spine

Calms the brain and helps alleviate stress and mild depression

Stimulates abdominal organs, lungs, and thyroid

Rejuvenates tired legs

Improves digestion

Helps relieve the symptoms of menopause

Relieves menstrual discomfort when done supported

Reduces anxiety, fatigue, backache, headache, and insomnia

Therapeutic for asthma, high blood pressure, osteoporosis, and
sinusitis

Use caution if you have a neck injury.

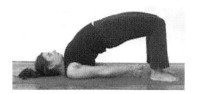

Lie supine on the floor, and if necessary, place a thickly folded blanket under your shoulders to protect your neck. Bend your knees and set your feet on the floor, heels as close to the sitting bones as possible.

Exhale and, pressing your inner feet and arms actively into the floor, push your tailbone upward toward the pubis, firming (but not hardening) the buttocks, and lift the buttocks off the floor. Keep your thighs and inner feet parallel. Clasp the hands below your pelvis and extend through the arms to help you stay on the tops of your shoulders.

Lift your buttocks until the thighs are about parallel to the floor. Keep your knees directly over the heels, but push them forward, away from the hips, and lengthen the tailbone toward the backs of the knees. Lift the pubis toward the navel.

Lift your chin slightly away from the sternum and, firming the shoulder blades against your back, press the top of the sternum toward the chin. Firm the outer arms, broaden the shoulder blades, and try to lift the space between them at the base of the neck (where it's resting on the blanket) up into the torso.

Stay in the pose anywhere from 30 seconds to 1 minute. Release with an exhalation, rolling the spine slowly down onto the floor.

Said to reverse the normal downward flow of a precious subtle fluid called amrita (immortal) or soma (extract) in the Hatha Yoga Pradipika, modern yogis agree that Viparita Karani may have the power to cure whatever ails you.

Benefits include:

Relieves tired or cramped legs and feet

Gently stretches the back legs, front torso, and the back of the neck

Relieves mild backache

Calms the mind

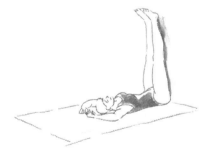

The pose described this is a passive, supported variation of the shoulder stand. For your support you'll need one or two thickly folded blankets or a firm round bolster. You'll also need to rest your legs vertically (or nearly so) on a wall or other upright support.

Before performing the pose, determine two things about your support: its height and its distance from the wall. If you're stiffer, the support should be lower and placed farther from the wall; if you're more flexible, use a higher support that is closer to the wall.

Your distance from the wall also depends on your height: if you're shorter move closer to the wall, if taller move farther from the wall. Experiment with the position of your support until you find the placement that works for you.

Start with your support about 5 to 6 inches away from the wall. Sit sideways on right end of the support, with your right side against the wall (left- handers can substitute "left" for "right" in these instructions). Exhale and, with one smooth movement, swing your legs up onto the wall and your shoulders and head lightly down onto the floor.

The first few times you do this you may slide off the support and plop down with your buttocks on the floor. Don't get discouraged. Try lowering the support and/or moving it slightly further off the wall until you gain some facility with this movement, then move back closer to the wall.

Your sitting bones don't need to be right against the wall, but they should be "dripping" down into the space between the support and the wall. Check that the front of your torso gently arches from the pubis to the top of the shoulders.

If the front of your torso seems flat, then you've probably slipped a bit off the support. Bend your knees, press your feet into the wall and lift your pelvis off the support a few inches, tuck the support a little higher up under your pelvis, then lower your pelvis onto the support again.

Lift and release the base of your skull away from the back of your neck and soften your throat. Don't push your chin against your sternum; instead let your sternum lift toward the chin. Take a small roll (made from a towel for example) under your neck if the cervical spine feels flat. Open your shoulder blades away from the spine and release your hands and arms out to your sides, palms up.

Keep your legs relatively firm, just enough to hold them vertically in place. Release the heads of the thigh bones and the weight of your belly deeply into your torso, toward the back of the pelvis. Soften your eyes and turn them down to look into your heart.

Stay in this pose anywhere from 5 to 15 minutes. Be sure not to twist off the support when coming out. Instead, slide off the support onto the floor before turning to the side.

You can also bend your knees and push your feet against the wall to lift your pelvis off the support. Then slide the support to one side, lower your pelvis to the floor, and turn to the side. Stay on your side for a few breaths, and come up to sitting with an exhalation.

CorpsePose-Savasana

Savasana is a pose of total relaxation—making it one of the most challenging asanas.

Benefits include:

Calms the brain and helps relieve stress and mild depression

Relaxes the body

Reduces headache, fatigue, and insomnia

Helps to lower blood pressure

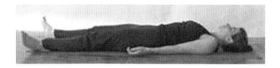

In Savasana it's essential that the body be placed in a neutral position. Sit on the floor with your knees bent, feet on the floor, and lean back onto your forearms. Lift your pelvis slightly off the floor and, with your hands, push the back of the pelvis toward the tailbone, then return the pelvis to the floor.

Inhale and slowly extend the right leg, then the left, pushing through the heels. Release both legs, softening the groins, and see that the legs are angled evenly relative to the mid-line of the torso, and that the feet turn out equally. You should narrow the front pelvis and soften (but don't flatten) the lower back.

With your hands lift the base of the skull away from the back of the neck and release the back of the neck down toward the tailbone. If you have any difficulty doing this, support the back of the head and neck on a folded blanket. Broaden the base of the skull too, and lift the crease of the neck diagonally into the center of the head. Make sure your ears are equidistant from your shoulders.

Reach your arms toward the ceiling, perpendicular to the floor. Rock slightly from side to side and broaden the back ribs and the shoulder blades away from the spine. Then release the arms to the floor, angled evenly relative to the mid-line of torso.

Turn the arms outward and stretch them away from the space between the shoulder blades. Rest the backs of the hands on the floor as close as you comfortably can to the index finger knuckles. Make sure the shoulder blades are resting evenly on the floor. Imagine the lower tips of the shoulder blades are lifting diagonally into your back toward the top of the sternum. From here, spread the collarbones.

In addition to quieting the physical body in Savasana, it's also necessary to pacify the sense organs. Soften the root of the tongue, the wings of the nose, the channels of the inner ears, and the skin of the forehead, especially around the bridge of the nose between the eyebrows. Let the eyes sink to the back of the head, then turn them downward to gaze at the heart. Release your brain to the back of the head.

Stay in this pose for 5 minutes for every 30 minutes of practice. To exit, first roll gently with an exhalation onto one side, preferably the right. Take 2 or 3 breaths. With another exhalation press your hands against the floor and lift your torso, dragging your head slowly after. The head should always come up last.

After completing these exercises, take a few moments to practice some deep meditation which is covered in the next section.

MEDITATION

Meditation can be more accurately called relaxation. It is striving to reach a state of serenity within your body and mind. Achieving a balance between the two can lead you to self-actualization and inner peace. Who couldn't use that?

Meditating is actually easier than you might imagine.

Most of us have probably dabbled in meditation by participating in conscious relaxation – perhaps during an exercise class or to manage pain at the dentist or anxiety before a test. We start by paying attention to our breathing. The practical effort of meditation is to focus completely on our breathing taking our minds away from the "mind clutter" that constantly tries to invade our mind and eliminates feelings that will lead to a time of calm.

With repeated effort the goal of clearing your mind – to think of nothing, does occur and the process of meditation takes on its own energy. The result is peace, serenity, calmness, eventually opening you to new insights.

Our world can be fast, fun and exciting. It is also challenging, trying, demanding and frightening. These two s i d e s of our l i v e s p r o d u c e stress, emotional reactions, anxiety, worry and anticipation. Our bodies and minds can tolerate only so much of any of these. After a while, each of us reaches a saturation point and the results become uncomfortable at best; for some it may be unbearable, even unendurable.

No magic pill is available to eliminate these feelings. The reality is, as the wise old man said, the answer is inside all of us. To manage these universal concerns we must go inside ourselves. Among the steps we can take is the learning and practicing of meditation.

There is no right or wrong behavior during your meditation. It is your time for you. Everyone deserves this kind of personal attention. This is a self-care activity; loving oneself!

Teach it to your children instead of a time-out in their room or corner. Teach it to your friends, family, anyone who will listen. We can share this gift and get back as we give. We are all better because of each person who meditates.

The peace and joy felt by those who meditate enters the world for all of us as positive energy. From it the world is a better place.

So what exactly is meditation?   There are many types of meditation. The one definition that fits almost all types is..."Consciously directing your attention to alter your state of consciousness."

There's no limit to the things you can direct your attention toward... symbols,   sounds,   colors,   breath,   uplifting thoughts, spiritual realms, etc.

Meditation is simply about attention... where you direct it, and how it alters your consciousness.

Traditionally meditation was (and still is) used for spiritual growth...i.e. becoming more conscious; unfolding our inner Light, Love, & Wisdom; becoming more aware of the guiding Presence in our lives; accelerating our journey home to our True Self... our Spirit.

More recently, meditation has become a valuable tool for finding a peaceful oasis of relaxation and stress relief in a demanding, fast-paced world.

It can be used for healing, emotional cleansing and balancing, deepening concentration, unlocking creativity, and finding inner guidance. Meditating is also the culmination of yoga exercises as your body reaches a state of relaxation, so should your mind.

When you begin your meditation, put your expectations aside, and don't worry about doing it right. There are infinite possibilities and no fixed criterion for determining right meditation. There are, however, a few things to avoid. Don't try to force something to happen. Don't over-analyze the meditation and don't try to make your mind blank or chase thoughts away. There is no one "right" way to meditate, so just concentrate on the process and find the best way for YOU!

Find a quiet, comfortable place to meditate. You can sit in a comfortable chair, on the bed, on the floor... anywhere that's comfortable. It's not necessary to sit cross-legged. Your legs can be in any position that is comfortable. Eliminate as much noise and as many potential distractions as possible. Don't worry about those things that you cannot control.

When you sit to meditate, sit comfortably, with your spine reasonably straight.
This allows the spiritual energy to flow freely up the spine, which is an important aspect of meditation. Leaning against a chair back, a wall, headboard, etc. is perfectly all right. If, for physical reasons, you can't sit up, lay flat on your back.

Place your hands in any position that is comfortable.

There are many types of meditation you can practice. We'll explore some of the more popular and effective ones.

UNIVERSALMANTRAMEDITATION

This meditation comes from an ancient Indian text called the Malini Vijaya Tantra, which dates back about 5000 years. It is a very easy meditation, yet very powerful in its capacity to quiet your mind and connect you with your Essence or Inner Spirit.

This meditation uses a mantra as your object of focus. A mantra is a word or phrase that has the power to catalyze a shift into deeper, more peaceful states of awareness. The mantra most use for this meditation is: Aum. Aum does not have a literal translation. Rather, it is the essential vibration of the universe. If you were to tune into the actual sound of the cosmos, the perpetual sound of Aummm is what you would hear.

Although this mantra is sometimes chanted aloud, in this meditation, you will be repeating the mantra mentally... silently. Before we get to the actual steps, there are a few important points to be aware of.

One of the keys to this meditation is repeating the mantra gently or faintly in your mind.

The power of this technique comes from letting go and allowing your attention to dive into the deeper realms of a w a r e n e s s . Therefore, even though you will be focusing on the mantra, staying focused on the mantra is not the aim of this meditation. Trying too hard to stay focused would keep your attention from descending into the deeper realms. Instead, you will be repeating the mantra with "minimal effort", and giving your mind the space to wander a bit.

Resist the temptation to make something happen, and allow the mantra to do the work.

This meditation easily produces a shift into deeper, more peaceful states of awareness. (The degree of this will vary from session to session.) It increases the flow of energy to the brain and clears away a good deal of physical and emotional toxins.

Because of this detoxification, it is best to keep this meditation to 10 or 15 minutes a day when first beginning. After a month or so, it can be increased to 20 minutes, but that should be the maximum for anyone who does not have quite a few years of meditation experience.
Also, it is advisable to drink a lot of pure water. Finally, mantra meditation accelerates spiritual growth as you achieve a state of relaxation and self-awareness.

1.   Sit comfortably, with your eyes closed and your spine reasonably straight.

2. Begin repeating the mantra gently in your mind.

3. Repeat the mantra at whatever tempo feels most natural. There is no need to synchronize the mantra with your breathing, but if this occurs naturally, it's ok.

4. Allow the mantra to arise more faintly in your mind... repeating it with minimal effort.

5. Continue repeating the mantra faintly, and allow for whatever happens.

6. If at any time, you feel that you are slipping into a sleep-like or dream-like state, allow it to happen.

7. If and when you notice that your attention has drifted completely off the mantra, gently begin repeating it again, and continue with minimal effort.

8. After 10 or 15 minutes, stop repeating the mantra, and come out of your meditation slowly.

RELAXATIONMEDITATION

This remarkably easy and relaxing meditation makes use of a little-known secret about the eyes. Allowing the eyes to rest in a soft downward gaze has an instant, automatic relaxing effect.

Relaxation meditation provides a great deal of stress reduction and can be used as a quick 2 minute relax and refresh break almost anywhere. You will also realize a heightened sense of alertness.

1. Sit comfortably with your spine reasonably straight.

2. Allow your eyes to rest comfortably downward, gazing softly, but not focused on anything.

3. Without closing your eyes completely, let your eyelids drop to a level that feels most comfortable.

4. Continue gazing downward... the act of gazing is your primary focus (rather than the area at which you are gazing). You may notice your breathing becoming more rhythmic.

5. It's ok to let your attention drift a bit. If your eyes become very heavy, it's ok to let them close. If you notice you've come out of your relaxed space, simply bring your attention back to your relaxed downward gaze.

ENERGYHEALINGMEDITATION

In this simple healing meditation, you send the powerful healing Life Force directly to the area in need of help. This Life Force is the energy behind all healing.

Wherever this energy is flowing and in balance, there is health and well-being. Wherever this energy is blocked or out of balance, illness manifests.

Many people believe in visualization as a key healing tool. Energy healing meditation helps you to concentrate your positive energy on an afflicted area and alleviate any adverse symptoms and feelings that are being manifested through the physical pain.

1. Sit reasonably straight and close your eyes.

2. Breathe slowly, as silently as possible. (Holding your breath after inhaling or exhaling is not recommended.)

3. As you inhale, feel yourself breathing the healing Life Force in through your solar plexus. Picture this Life Force as a very refined, light energy.

4. As you exhale, gently direct this light energy to the afflicted area. If there is not a specific ailing area, disperse this light energy throughout your body as you exhale.

5. Continue until you feel the area has received enough Life Force.

COLORHEALINGMEDITATION

We are not just our physical selves.

We are multi-dimensional beings, composed of an Inner Spirit, a mental body, an emotional body, a vital body, and a physical body. The energy of these bodies becomes progressively subtler from physical to spiritual. Illness begins with disharmony in one of these energy bodies. If not harmonized, the disease moves outward, affecting the denser bodies, ultimately manifesting as physical illness.

Total healing requires restoring harmony to all of our bodies. This meditation is designed to cleanse and harmonize your various bodies with the healing energies of color.

Color healing meditation will provide you with cleansing, balancing, & healing at all levels: Spiritual, Mental, Emotional, Vital, & Physical. It also will develop concentration & visualization abilities.

1. Sit comfortably with your eyes closed.

2. Visualize a large ball of radiant Golden light a few inches over your head.

Visualize that ball of light slowly descending through your crown, filling your entire being with golden light.

3. Imagine yourself absorbing that light as it nourishes, cleanses & heals your whole being - your Spirit and all of your bodies - dissolving all blocked and toxic energies.

4. Repeat this exercise, visualizing a ball of Red light. Continue through the entire spectrum like this, visualizing a ball of Orange light; Yellow light; Green light; Blue light; Indigo light; and Violet light. Go through the spectrum at whatever pace feels appropriate.

5. Take some time to visualize yourself in a state of perfect, radiant health.

CENTERING

Centering is meditation in action. Within you is a space that is always calm and at peace. This space is often referred to as your "calm center". Being centered means remaining in your calm center amidst the busyness of everyday life. Being centered means not allowing your inner light to be overshadowed by stressful circumstances or negative thoughts and emotions.

When you are centered, you are in a state of clarity, focus, peace, and balance. When you are not centered, you are unclear, unfocussed, stressed, and off balance.

A good centering technique will require only minimal attention, allowing you to keep some of your attention on the activity at hand. Here are some very easy, effective centering techniques.

1. Simple Breath Awareness

While involved in whatever you are doing, bring some attention to your breathing for just a few moments... it needn't be your full attention... just enough to bring you back to your calm center. Breathe naturally, or perhaps just a little more slowly and deeply.

2. Reclaiming Your Energy

When you are feeling stressed and scattered, take several slow, deep breaths. With each in-breath, imagine you are pulling all of your scattered energy and attention back to your inner self... your calm center.

3. Letting Go

This centering technique combines breath awareness with the phrase or mantra, "Let go." It is especially helpful when you are tense and/or fixating on a stressful situation or a negative thought or emotion. As you inhale, (silently or aloud) say, "Let"
As you exhale, say "go"... while letting go of all that is stressing you.

4. Inner Sun

Imagine a bright sun filling your heart chakra... the calm, subtle energy field that permeates your chest area. Imagine that sun gently emanating peace and joy throughout your entire being.

Yoga and meditation certainly have proven to be effective tools to lessen stress and provide a sense of calm that cannot be achieved through conventional exercise. So what about those stress-filled days at the office when you are unable to concentrate on work because of outside distractions? You can perform yoga right at your desk if you want! Let's look at "desktop yoga".

DESKTOP YOGA

Whether you're a high-powered executive or an administrative assistant with your boss's problems becoming your own, many people in the business world experience an inordinate amount of stress at the office. It would be nice to have a quiet place to practice conventional yoga techniques, but that isn't always possible.

Yoga experts have devised a way for you to do a short yoga program right at your desk. Try these exercises to de-stress at the office.

Sit up tall in your chair, or if possible stand up. Stretch your arms overhead and interlock your fingers, turn the palms to the ceiling. Take a deep breathe in and on the exhale extend your side torso and take the tips of the shoulder blades into the body. Take another deep breathe and on the exhale stretch to the right, inhale come up and exhale stretch to the left.

On an inhale, lift your shoulders up to your ears and then exhale and let them drop. Repeat 3 times. Contract the shoulder muscle fully when you lift your shoulders up and then on the drop it will release more completely.

Stand (or sit at your desk) with your feet planted firmly in the ground. Inhale and raise the arms out to the side, palms down. Exhale and rotate the palms up, rolling the shoulders back. Take an inhale and on the exhale, bend the elbows in toward the waist. Inhale and on the exhale bring the palms to the belly. This exercise helps to open the chest and extend the upper back.

Take your hands behind your back and interlock the fingers, stretching the shoulders back, opening the chest. Take several breaths. Make sure that your head stays in the mid-line and that your eye gaze is on the horizon.

Stand by the wall, extend your right arm and place the palm on the wall with the fingers up. On an exhale, turn your chest away, taking the shoulder blade into the torso.

Stand by your desk and place your palms on the desk top with the fingers pointing toward your body. Gently stretch the lower arm and wrist.

Wrap the right arm around the torso and place your right hand on the left shoulder with the elbow at chest height and facing forward.

Put your left hand on the right elbow and on an exhale, stretch it toward the left, opening between the shoulder blades. Hold for several breaths and then release. Repeat on the other side

Reach the right arm into the air and on an exhale bend the elbow and reach your fingers down the back, between the shoulder blades. Place the left hand on the elbow and on an exhale gently pull the elbow to the left. Relax the ribs and hold for several breaths. Release and repeat on the other side

Hug your arms around your chest and then put one elbow underneath the other, the hand facing toward each other and fingers to the ceiling. Exhale and slowly raise the arms so that the elbows come up to the height of the shoulder, keep the shoulders down. Repeat on the other side.

Sit on your chair and pull back away from the desk, resting your palms on the desk top and extend your side torso.
Lift the ribs up, let the shoulder blades slide towards the desk, and make sure the head is extended from the spine with the chin towards the chest.

Sit on your chair, feet planted firmly in the floor, sitting bones pressing into the chair. Extend the side torso, and twist to the right (on an exhale), one hand on back to chair, one hand on the side of the chair. Hold for a few breaths and then repeat the other side.

Sit forward on your chair and open the legs a little wider than the hips. Lean forward from the hips and drop your torso down. Let the head and arms hang down toward the floor.

Sit upright in your chair with your feet planted firmly on the ground. Press your sitting bones down into the chair and extend the side torso. Relax your shoulders. Place your palms on your knees and spread the fingers wide. Take a deep breath in and on the exhale extend your tongue to your chin; focus your eyes to your nose. Inhale and bring the tongue back into the mouth. Exhale and stick the tongue out again and this time focus the eyes up to your forehead. Repeat 3 times.

Sit upright on chair, relax your shoulders and extend the side torso up. Relax your facial muscles, the jaw and tongue. Circle the eyes clockwise 8 times and counter-clockwise 8 times. Close your eyes and breathe deeply for a few slow breaths.
You may want to try a quick relaxation meditation to wrap up this session just as a way to refresh and regroup.

Yoga can be used for more than simple de-stressing. It can also be used to alleviate the symptoms of everyday ailments without the use of medication.

YOGA FOR HEADACHES

There are many different kinds of headaches. Some (like tension headaches and migraines) are fairly common; others (like sinus headaches or headaches caused by brain tumors) are relatively rare. Various treatments are recommended for dealing with headaches. Yoga asanas and breathing can help too, though mostly with tension-type headaches.

Everyone gets a tension headache now and again, but if you suffer from this type of headache habitually, it's important to consult a doctor or other health practitioner to treat the pain and work to resolve the ultimate source of the tension.

When treating a tension headache with asanas and breathing, it's important to start practicing as soon as possible after you start to feel the pain. Once the headache is established it will be very difficult to alleviate.

Here are the yoga positions that can be used to alleviate a headache: Child'sPose(Balasana)

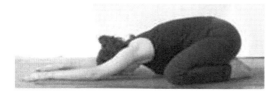

1. Kneel on the floor. Touch your big toes together and sit on your heels, then separate your knees about as wide as your hips.

2. Exhale and lay your torso down between your thighs. Broaden your sacrum across the back of your pelvis and

narrow your hip points toward the navel, so that they nestle down onto the inner thighs. Lengthen your tailbone away from the back of the pelvis while you lift the base of your skull away from the back of your neck.

3. Lay your hands on the floor alongside your torso, palms up, and release the fronts of your shoulders toward the floor. Feel how the weight of the front shoulders pulls the shoulder blades wide across your back.

4. Balasana is a resting pose. Stay anywhere from 30 seconds to a few minutes. Beginners can also use Balasana to get a taste of a deep forward bend, where the torso rests on the thighs. Stay in the pose from 1 to 3 minutes. To come up, first lengthen the front torso, and then with an inhalation lift from the tailbone as it presses down and into the pelvis.

Note: you can do the child's pose when you get tired, out of breath, or need to rest.
Simply pick up with your exercises again when refreshed. Child's pose is also a great way to quickly alleviate stress at any time.

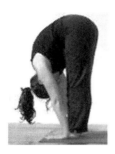

1.   Stand in relaxed position with your hands on your hips. Exhale and bend forward from the hip joints, not from the waist. As you descend draw the front torso out of the groins and open the space between the pubis and top sternum. As in all the forward bends, the emphasis is on lengthening the front torso as you move more fully into the position.

2.   If possible, with your knees straight, bring your palms or finger tips to the floor slightly in front of or beside your feet, or bring your palms to the backs of your ankles. If this isn't possible, cross your forearms and hold your elbows. Press the heels firmly into the floor and lift the sitting bones toward the ceiling. Turn the top thighs slightly inward.

3.   With each inhalation in the pose, lift and lengthen the front torso just slightly; with each exhalation release a little more fully into the forward bend. In this way the torso oscillates almost imperceptibly with the breath.

Let your head hang from the root of the neck, which is deep in the upper back, between the shoulder blades.

4.   This pose can be used as a resting position between the standing poses. Stay in the pose for 30 seconds to 1 minute.

It can also be practiced as a pose in itself.

5. Don't roll the spine to come up. Instead bring your hands back onto your hips and reaffirm the length of the front torso. Then press your tailbone down and into the pelvis and come up on an inhalation with a long front torso.

YOGA FOR MENSTRUAL CRAMPS

Menstrual cramps can be very debilitating for those who suffer from severe cramps early in their cycle. While your first inclination might be to lay on your couch in the fetus position moaning in pain, try yoga to relieve the pain.

Exercise during menstruation is generally highly recommended. It's believed that exercise can ease the discomfort of your period; quell mood swings, anxiety, and depression; and reduce bloating.

Most contemporary yoga teachers advise a fairly conservative approach toward asana practice during menstruation. This makes perfect sense for women who feel sluggish during their cycle.
However, many other women don't feel the need to change anything about their practice during menstruation, except maybe to limit strenuous inverted poses. Each student should decide for herself what kind of asana sequence is most appropriate for her body during menstruation.

RecliningBoundAngle

Sit with the soles of your feet touching each other. Exhale and lower your back torso toward the floor, first leaning on your hands.

Once you are leaning back on your forearms, use your hands to spread the back of your pelvis and release your lower back and upper buttocks through your tailbone. Bring your torso all the way to the floor, supporting your head and neck on a blanket roll or bolster if needed.

With your hands grip your topmost thighs and rotate your inner thighs externally, pressing your outer thighs away from the sides of your torso. Next slide your hands along your outer thighs from the hips toward the knees and widen your outer knees away from your hips.

Then slide your hands down along your inner thighs, from the knees to the groins. Imagine that your inner groins are sinking into your pelvis. Push your hip points together, so that while the back pelvis widens, the front pelvis narrows.

Lay your arms on the floor, angled at about 45 degrees from the sides of your torso, palms up.

The natural tendency in this pose is to push the knees toward the floor in the belief that this will increase the stretch of the inner thighs and groins. But especially if your groins are tight, pushing the knees down will have just the opposite of the intended effect: The groins will harden, as will your belly and lower back. Instead, imagine that your knees are floating up toward the ceiling and continue settling your groins deep into your pelvis. As your groins drop toward the floor, so will your knees.

To start, stay in this pose for one minute. Gradually extend your stay anywhere from five to 10 minutes. To come out, use your hands to press your thighs together, then roll over onto one side and push yourself away from the floor, head trailing the torso.

Move back into sitting position with the soles of your feet touching

UpwardBow

Basically, this is a simple back bend. Lay on the floor, place your hands above your head flat on the floor and raise your back into an arched position.

SeatedTwist

Still sitting twist to the right with an exhalation, hold for 30 seconds, then twist to the left for 30 seconds. Repeat three times to each side, each time holding for 30 seconds.

YOGA FOR DEPRESSION

The word "depression" covers a wide range of conditions, from long- standing and severe clinical or major depression to shorter-term and episodic mild depression, to situational depression brought on by a major life change, such as the death of a spouse, job loss, divorce.

Many different therapies are available for depression, including anti- depressants and psychotherapy. Studies indicate that regular exercise too, including yoga asanas and breathing, can help some people ease the symptoms of mild to moderate forms of depression.

Of course, one major hurdle in using exercise to alleviate depression is motivation, or lack of it.

Most depressed people don't really feel much like getting out of bed in the morning, much less exercising.

Then too, failure to see the exercise program through can make a depressed person feel even worse.

So start off slowly, and be sure to choose an exercise that you really enjoy; if possible, exercise with a supportive partner or group. Try to exercise at least three times a week.

Reclining Bound Angle – Downward Facing Dog – Standing ForwardBend– Headstand

Use a folded blanket or sticky mat to pad your head and forearms. Kneel on the floor. Lace your fingers together and set the forearms on the floor, elbows at shoulder width.

Roll the upper arms slightly outward, but press the inner wrists firmly into the floor. Set the crown of your head on the floor.

If you are just beginning to practice this pose, press the bases of your palms together and snuggle the back of your head against the clasped hands. More experienced students can open their hands and place the back of the head into the open palms.

Inhale and lift your knees off the floor. Carefully walk your feet closer to your elbows, heels elevated. Actively lift through the top thighs, forming an inverted "V."

Firm the shoulder blades against your back and lift them toward the tailbone so the front torso stays as long as possible. This should help prevent the weight of the shoulders collapsing onto your neck and head.

Exhale and lift your feet away from the floor. Take both feet up at the same time, even if it means bending your knees and hopping lightly off the floor. As the legs (or thighs, if your knees are bent) rise to perpendicular to the floor, firm the tailbone against the back of the pelvis.

Turn the upper thighs in slightly, and actively press the heels toward the ceiling (straightening the knees if you bent them to come up). The center of the arches should align over the center of the pelvis, which in turn should align over the crown of the head.

Firm the outer arms inward, and soften the fingers. Continue to press the shoulder blades against the back, widen them, and draw them toward the tailbone. Keep the weight evenly balanced on the two forearms.

It's also essential that your tailbone continues to lift upward toward the heels. Once the backs of the legs are fully lengthened through the heels, maintain that length and press up through the balls of the big toes so the inner legs are slightly longer than the outer.

As a beginner, stay in this position for 10 seconds. Gradually add 5 to 10 seconds onto your stay every day or so until you can comfortably hold the pose for 3 minutes. Then continue for 3 minutes each day for a week or two, until you feel relatively comfortable in the pose.

Again gradually add 5 to 10 seconds onto your stay every day or so until you can comfortably hold the pose for 5 minutes. Come down with an exhalation, without losing the lift of the shoulder blades, with both feet touching the floor at the same time.

Upward Bow– SeatedTwist– Bridge–
HeadtoKneeForwardBend

Benefits Include:

Calms the brain and helps relieve mild depression Stretches the spine, shoulders, hamstrings, and groins Stimulates the liver and kidneys
Improves digestion

Helps relieve the symptoms of menopause

Relieves anxiety, fatigue, headache, menstrual discomfort

Therapeutic for high blood pressure, insomnia, and sinusitis

Strengthens the back muscles during pregnancy (up to second trimester), done without coming forward, keeping your back spine concave and front torso long.

Use caution with this pose if you have a knee injury.

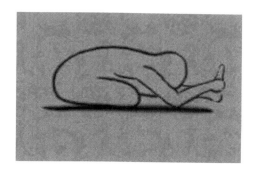

1. Sit on the floor with your buttocks lifted on a folded blanket and your legs straight in front of you. Inhale, bend your right knee, and draw the heel back toward your perineum. Rest your right foot sole lightly against your inner left thigh, and lay the outer right leg on the floor, with the shin at a right angle to the left leg (if your right knee doesn't rest comfortably on the floor, support it with a folded blanket).

2. Press your right hand against the inner right groin, where the thigh joins the pelvis, and your left hand on the floor beside the hip.

Exhale and turn the torso slightly to the left, lifting the torso as you push down on and

ground the inner right thigh. Line up your navel with the middle of the left thigh. You can just stay here, using a strap to help you lengthen the spine evenly, grounding through the sitting bones.

3. Or, when you are ready, you can drop the strap and reach out with your right hand to take the inner left foot, thumb on the sole. Inhale and lift the front torso, pressing the top of the left thigh into the floor and extending actively through the left heel. Use the pressure of the left hand on the floor to increase the twist to the left. Then reach your left hand to the outside of the foot. With the arms fully extended, lengthen the front torso from the pubis to the top of the sternum.

4. Exhale and extend forward from the groins, not the hips. Be sure not to pull yourself forcefully into the forward bend, hunching the back and shortening the front torso. As you descend, bend your elbows out to the sides and lift them away from the floor.

5. Lengthen forward into a comfortable stretch. The lower belly should touch the thighs first, the head last. Stay in the pose anywhere from 1 to 3 minutes. Come up with an inhalation and repeat the instructions with the legs reversed for the same length of time.

CONCLUSION

The popularity of yoga is, without a doubt, increasing as people are constantly trying to balance the stresses of everyday life with their own spiritual well-being.

It is important for you, the reader, to realize that we are not medical professionals and have simply tried to provide you with an introduction to yoga and meditation. This book is a way for you to get started on your own yoga program.

If you have special health considerations, you should be sure and consult with your doctor before embarking on a yoga program, or any other exercise program for that matter. We cannot be held responsible in any way for any problems that may arise from your yoga journey. This is meant simply as an informational tool to help you start down that path.

But you will find that once you start initiating yoga into your daily exercise routine, you will most likely notice a heightened state of well-being and a more spiritual connection to both your inner self as well as any higher power you choose to acknowledge.

Remember to concentrate on your breathing when performing the poses, and don't force your body into positions it isn't comfortable doing. When meditating, focus on the inner calm you are trying to achieve.

Perform these exercises when you get the chance. You don't have to do a full cycle to feel better. Even practicing one exercise when you have the time can have huge therapeutic benefits to mind, body, and soul!

Yoga can better your life in so many ways. It can help you become a better spouse, parent, worker, and person. You can help others by spreading your experiences with yoga and meditation. Imagine the thanks you'll receive as you tell others how this ancient art has enhanced your life!

Shanti (peace) to you as you journey to your own Shambhala (place of utter tranquility).

To show your appreciation to the author and help others have wonderful reading experiences and find helpful information too, we'd be very grateful if you'd kindly

COPYRIGHT INFORMATION

DISCLAIMER AND TERMS OF USE

This information is not presented by a medical practitioner and is for educational and informational purposes only. The content is not intended to be a substitute for professional medical advice, diagnosis, or treatment. Always seek the advice of your physician or other qualified health provider with any questions you may have regarding a medical condition. Never disregard professional medical advice or delay in seeking it because of something you have read.

Since natural and/or dietary supplements are not FDA approved, they must be accompanied by a two-part disclaimer on the product label: that the statement has not been evaluated by FDA and that the product is not intended to "diagnose, treat, cure or prevent any disease.

The author and publisher of this course and the accompanying materials have used their best efforts in preparing this course. The author and publisher make no representation or warranties with respect to the accuracy, applicability, fitness, or completeness of the contents of this course. The information contained in this course is strictly for educational purposes. Therefore, if you wish to apply ideas contained in this course, you are taking full responsibility for your actions.

The author and publisher disclaim any warranties (express or implied), merchantability, or fitness for any particular purpose. The author and publisher shall in no event be held liable to any party for any direct, indirect, punitive, special, incidental or other consequential damages arising directly or indirectly from any use of this material, which is provided "as is", and without warranties.

As always, the advice of a competent legal, tax, accounting, medical or other professional should be sought. The author and publisher do not warrant the performance, effectiveness or applicability of any sites listed or linked to in this course.

All links are for information purposes only and are not warranted for content, accuracy or any other implied or explicit purpose.

This report is © Copyrighted by PlayMore Publishing. No part of this may be copied, or changed in any format, or used in any way other than what is outlined within this course under any circumstances. Violators would be prosecuted severely.

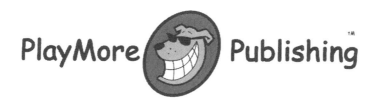

3788919R00047

Printed in Great Britain
by Amazon.co.uk, Ltd.,
Marston Gate.